Th Workouts
To Burn Fat, Tone Up and Lose Weight
By Dale L. Roberts
©2015

The 11 Best Cardio Workouts To Burn Fat, Tone Up, and Lose Weight
All rights reserved
ISBN-13: 978-1519414472
ISBN-10: 1519414471
April 5, 2015
Copyright ©2015 One Jacked Monkey, LLC
All photos courtesy of Dale L. Roberts, January 2015
No part of this book may be reproduced or transmitted in any form or by any means, electronic or mechanical, including photocopying, recording or by any information storage and retrieval system, without the permission in writing from One Jacked Monkey, LLC.

DISCLAIMER

This book proposes a program of exercise recommendations. However, all readers must consult a qualified medical professional before starting this or any other health & fitness program. As with any exercise program, if at any time you experience any discomfort, pain or duress of any sort, stop immediately and consult your physician. This book is intended for an audience that is free of any health condition, physical limitation or injury. The creators, producers, participants, advertisers and distributors of this program disclaim any liabilities or losses in connection with the exercises or advice herein. Any equipment or workout area that is used should be thoroughly inspected ahead of use as free of danger, flaw or compromise. The user assumes all responsibility when performing any movements contained in this book and waives the equipment manufacturer, makers and distributors of the equipment of all liabilities.

Table of Contents

Introduction 1
General Cardio Guidelines 5
The Four Treadmill Change-Up Routines 8
    Part 1.1: Treadmill Change-up 11
    Part 1.2: Treadmill Change-up 12
    Part 1.3: Treadmill Change-up 14
    Part 1.4: Treadmill Change-up 16
The Four Elliptical Whippin' Routines 18
    Part 2.1: Elliptical Whippin' 21
    Part 2.2: Elliptical Whippin' 22
    Part 2.3: Elliptical Whippin' 24
    Part 2.4: Elliptical Whippin' 26
The Four Break-a-bike Routines 28
    Part 3.1: Break-a-bike 30
    Part 3.2: Break-a-bike 31
    Part 3.3: Break-a-bike 32
Conclusion 34
Thank You.. 37
About The Author 38
Special Thanks... 39
ATTENTION: Get Your Free Gift 40
References 41

Introduction

Benjamin Franklin once said that "in this world nothing can be said to be certain, except death and taxes."[i] Yet, with tongue-in-cheek, I wholeheartedly disagree and add a third exception in cardio-respiratory training or better known as cardio. After all, most everyone who looks to get into great shape try what others have tried before them. Running, power walking, biking, stair climbing and other activities are what people use to get their cardio fix. But, why exactly are they doing cardio?

In early-2015, the World Health Organization (W.H.O.) stated that over 1.9 billion adults were overweight and 600 million of them were obese. The W.H.O. reported that in 2014, a staggering 39% of adults were overweight and 13% were obese. [ii] So, it's no surprise that eventually a portion of the overweight population look for a solution to relieve them of their unwanted bodyweight. And, in some instances, their family physician may vaguely suggest exercise or cardio. Well, where do they start? And, do they have to put in grueling hours at the gym?

In my opinion, cardio-respiratory training should not be optional in fitness training, it should be mandatory. Overlooking this area of health and fitness is like avoiding dental care. Teeth are important in eating and proper digestion. So, losing teeth impedes eating and digestion. That's why tooth brushing, flossing, and mouth washing exists—to protect your health. And, that is the parallel between oral care and cardio.

Simply put, cardio is for strengthening and building endurance in the cardio-respiratory system, collectively the heart and the lungs. The heart is a muscle and much like any other muscle in the body, deserves time, attention, and diligent training in your weight loss plans. When you train your heart, you gain stamina, endurance, and energy. Cardio training makes everyday tasks and living much easier, from your workouts to the most mundane chore. And, the best part is that cardio is appropriate for most everyone.

If boredom is your excuse to avoid cardio training at the gym, then I have your solution. I'm a bit different from other personal trainers and lean a little more on lower impact alternatives due to my experience in working with overweight clients, senior citizens, and special needs populations. These types of clients need to have something that will be effective yet safe on their joints, so I devise these programs to suit most anyone.

Though I have developed low-impact cardio programming, as per usual, please consult your family doctor for prior approval. These routines may NOT be appropriate for you and even if we had a one-on-one training consultation, I'd still require this prior to your start.

The first thing you will notice is the use of intervals throughout each of these programs. Gone are the days of trudging along at the same pace for minutes at a time. It has been proven time and again that high-intensity interval

The 11 Best Cardio Workouts

training burns more calories and trains the heart better than the traditional cardio sessions that are prolonged medium-to-low effort or intensity.[iii]

The book is split up into three types of equipment—treadmill, elliptical, and recumbent bike. Not all cardio equipment is the same so you may have to adjust the levels you do to match the equipment you use. Some programs may transfer to other cardio equipment. For example, you can substitute the recumbent bike for an upright bike. Or, use the elliptical programming on various other models. Use your best judgment when you workout.

Your efforts should be intense with heavy breathing and having little ability to talk. On a scale of 0-10, 0 being no exertion and 10 being completely breathless, you should be between 6-8 rating. The scale is entirely subjective, so don't compare your efforts with anyone else. Stay honest and continually re-evaluate your work with every exercise and workout. Avoid exercising at an intensity of 10, because this can be detrimental to your health and you should never push yourself until you cannot breathe properly. At lower intensity levels, enjoy the rest and recovery before you jump into the next intense burst. The rest is just as important as the harder efforts.

The bottom line is the concept of intervals allows me to create cardio programming that is far from the average cardio session. Stop worrying over the graphs and charts you find on equipment. Throw out the pre-programmed insane routines the cardio equipment companies provide you. This book is your golden ticket to less boring cardio routines and better cardio workouts. Now, read on, dig in, and have fun with your cardio for a change!

The 11 Best Cardio Workouts

General Cardio Guidelines

(This contains an excerpt from *The 3 Keys to Greater Health & Happiness*)

If you want to get the most out of your cardio workouts or resistance training, it is crucial for you to know where your heart rate is at during your efforts. Keep an eye on how much your heart rate elevates with each increase in level or intensity on the equipment. In the conclusion, I discuss two different options for monitoring your heart rate. The cheapest solution to checking your pulse is on your radial artery in your wrist. Practice pulse checking prior to working out so that you have a firm grasp on finger placement. American Heart Association is a great resource for proper pulse checking.

For anyone with special conditions, health needs or are taking prescribed medication, consult your doctor on the safest heart rate for your cardio training. Based on the complexity of your situation, you need a doctor-prescribed heart rate range that is safe and effective. With practice in fitness, your doctor will adjust your training level with time and consistent exercise.

Cardio training is considered exercising the heart at 50-85% of maximum heart rate (MHR) or maximum beats per minute. I'll discuss the relevance of the percentage of maximum heart rate a little later. First, you must know your maximum heart rate to stay safe. Training between 50-85% of your maximum heart rate puts enough stress on your heart to build strength and endurance while burning calories. No need to work too hard, because this can be counterproductive to your goals and destructive to your body.

Harvard Men's Health Watch published a recent study by Colorado scientists that revealed a formula that closely estimates maximum heart rate:[iv]

maximum heart rate = 208 - (0.7 x age in years)

Based on this formula, here is a chart to help with maximum heart rate (MHR) relevant to age and the heart beats per minute needed for minimum and maximum guidelines for cardio training:

Age	MHR	50%	70 - 85%
20	194	97	136 - 165
25	191	95	134 - 162
30	187	93	131 - 159
35	184	92	129 - 156
40	180	90	126 - 153
45	177	88	124 - 150
50	173	86	119 - 147
55	170	85	115 - 140
60	166	83	111 – 135
65	163	81	107 – 130

The lower intensity of 50% MHR is for someone who is just starting a fitness routine. If you find it too easy at 50% MHR, then increase your MHR by 5% to see how you handle that intensity. Gradually over the course of 3-4 weeks, work your way up towards the higher intensity. It's okay if you don't get to 70-85% MHR in one month. In due time and consistent cardio exercise, you will train your heart to handle higher intensity levels.

The higher intensity of 70-85% MHR is ideal for someone who is experienced in exercise. If you are new to exercise, this should be a big goal for you to achieve.

Dale L. Roberts

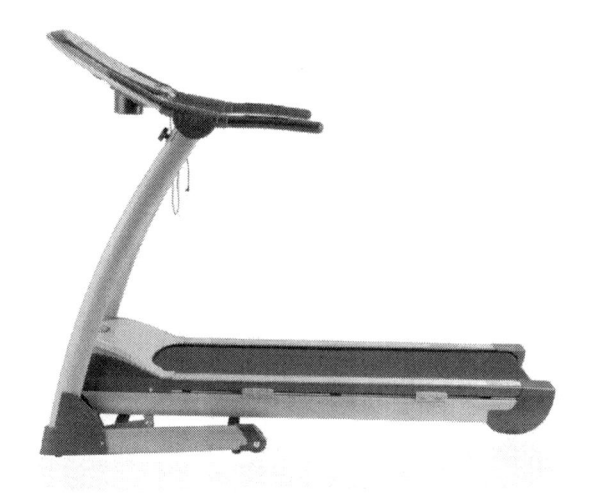

The Four Treadmill Change-Up Routines

This chapter is a four-part cardio series dedicated to the treadmill. The routines are in order of difficulty, so master the first program before moving onto the next. The equipment doesn't have to be fancy. Just use an average treadmill with incline capabilities for this cardio routine.

Always warm-up for a minimum of 5 minutes prior to any workout routine—whether weights, running, cardio or any other physically challenging activity. Warming up is not just for show or a waste of your time. It's for priming up the pump, greasing the gears and getting your body in optimal condition to begin maximizing the most out of every movement.

Please remember that for best results, holding onto the treadmill is discouraged in this routine. If you are unable to use a treadmill without a death grip on the machine, then you should not use this program. Remember, most treadmills are equipped with an emergency shut-off that you can pin to your clothes. People humble themselves by falling off a treadmill, so spare yourself the embarrassment and put the safety clip on in case you fall.

It's important to push yourself and hold yourself accountable, but never sacrifice good form, and proper cadence. Keep your posture erect, arms swinging forward and backward with each stride and use the safety clip on the treadmill when you need to have a safety stop feature. Cadence is the pace you walk according to the treadmill speed. Don't go faster than you can handle. If you find that 3.5 mph is too fast, then slow the treadmill to a manageable speed. The incline feature makes it difficult enough, so gauge what works best for you and adjust accordingly.

You will break a sweat on these cardio workouts, so come equipped with a large bottle of water, a workout towel, and firm resolve to complete this routine.

The 11 Best Cardio Workouts

Part 1.1: Treadmill Change-up

MINUTES	SPEED	INCLINE
0-5 Warm-up	3.5	0
5-6	3.5	1.5
6-7	3.5	3.0
7-8	3.5	4.5
8-9	3.5	6.0
9-10	3.5	7.5
10-11	3.5	9.0
11-12	3.5	10.5
12-13	3.5	12.0
13-14	3.5	13.5
14-15	3.5	15.0
15-16	3.5	13.0
16-17	3.5	14.0
17-18	3.5	12.0
18-19	3.5	13.0
19-20	3.5	11.0
20-21	3.5	12.0
21-22	3.5	10.0
22-23	3.5	11.0
23-24	3.5	9.0
24-25	3.5	10.0
25-26	3.5	8.0
26-30 Cooldown	3.5	5.0

Part 1.2: Treadmill Change-up

Assuming you completed the first part of the *Treadmill Change-up* series, this second part is an excellent progression to spice up your routine in the gym. The ever-increasing incline will leave you breathless quickly. Do not progress to this routine until you master the *Part 1.1 of the Treadmill Change-up* routines.

The 11 Best Cardio Workouts

MINUTES	SPEED	INCLINE
0-5 Warm-up	3.5	5.0
5-6	3.5	7.0
6-7	3.5	6.0
7-8	3.5	8.0
8-9	3.5	7.0
9-10	3.5	9.0
10-11	3.5	8.0
11-12	3.5	10.0
12-13	3.5	9.0
13-14	3.5	11.0
14-15	3.5	10.0
15-16	3.5	12.0
16-17	3.5	11.0
17-18	3.5	13.0
18-19	3.5	12.0
19-20	3.5	14.0
20-21	3.5	13.0
21-22	3.5	15.0
22-23	3.5	14.0
23-24	3.5	12.0
24-25	3.5	13.0
25-26	3.5	11.0
26-30 Cooldown	3.5	5.0

Part 1.3: Treadmill Change-up

I hope you have been progressing well in this four-part treadmill series. If you haven't yet mastered the past two routines, then just review this next cardio template and hold off until you are 100% confident and ready to complete it.

I changed the speed this time so the pace could be too fast for people with shorter strides. If that is the case, adjust the speed where appropriate and use your best judgment. Having a challenge is one thing, but creating adversity is altogether different. Be safe and have fun with this routine.

Time to get this new routine and OWN IT:

The 11 Best Cardio Workouts

MINUTES	SPEED	INCLINE
0-5 Warm-up	3.5	5.0
5-6	4.5	0.0
6-7	4.4	1.0
7-8	4.3	2.0
8-9	4.2	3.0
9-10	4.1	4.0
10-11	4.0	5.0
11-12	3.9	7.0
12-13	3.8	9.0
13-14	3.7	11.0
14-15	3.6	13.0
15-16	3.5	15.0
16-17	3.6	14.0
17-18	3.7	12.0
18-19	3.8	10.0
19-20	3.9	8.0
20-21	4.0	6.0
21-22	4.1	4.0
22-23	4.2	3.0
23-24	4.3	2.0
24-25	4.4	1.0
25-26	4.5	0.0
26-30 Cooldown	3.5	5.0

Part 1.4: Treadmill Change-up

This is the final part of the *Treadmill Change-up* series. As per usual, if you have not mastered the previous low-impact treadmill routines, then chances are unlikely you may not safely complete this routine. I encourage you to push yourself and grow by the day, but not at the detriment of your physical safety and health. This routine is no joke, so proceed with more caution than you have before. For those of you with the experience and the intestinal fortitude, progress forward.

The 11 Best Cardio Workouts

MINUTES	SPEED	INCLINE
0-5 Warm-up	3.5	5.0
5-6	3.5	15.0
6-7	3.5	1.0
7-8	3.6	14.0
8-9	3.6	2.0
9-10	3.7	13.0
10-11	3.7	3.0
11-12	3.8	12.0
12-13	3.8	4.0
13-14	3.9	11.0
14-15	3.9	5.0
15-16	4.0	10.0
16-17	4.0	6.0
17-18	4.1	9.0
18-19	4.1	7.0
19-20	4.2	8.0
20-21	4.2	9.0
21-22	4.3	10.0
22-23	4.3	11.0
23-24	4.4	12.0
24-25	4.4	13.0
25-26	4.5	14.0
26-30 Cooldown	3.5	5.0

Dale L. Roberts

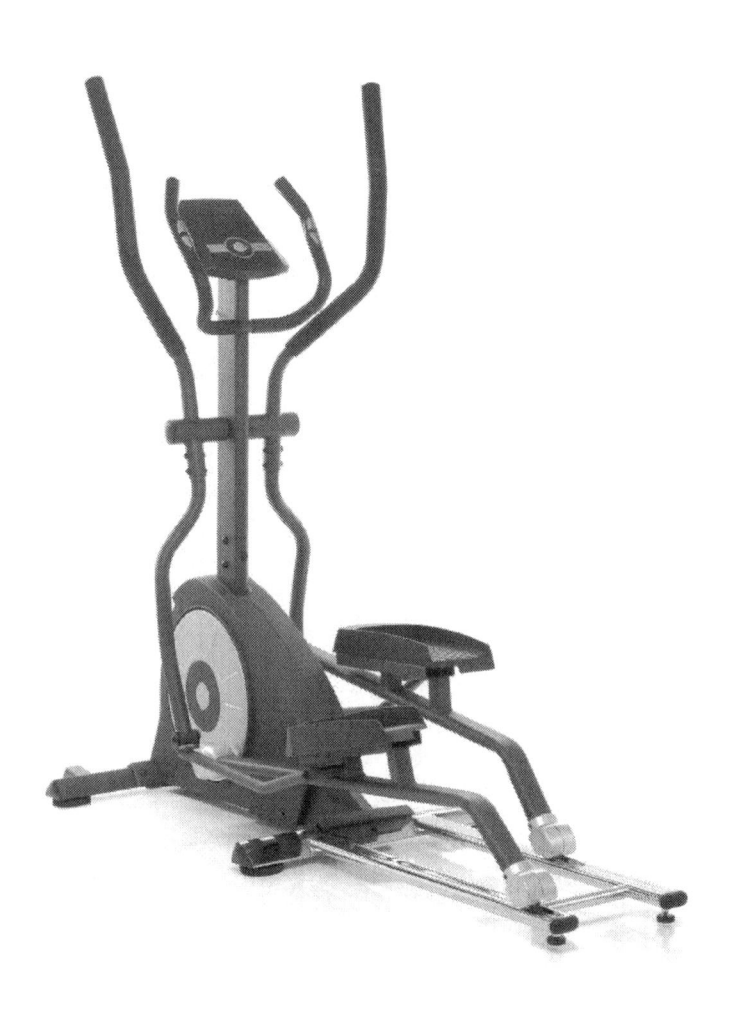

The Four Elliptical Whippin' Routines

I hope you found some great value in the four-part low-impact treadmill series. Not one to disappoint, I whipped together some more interesting cardio routines that will train your heart and give you an explosion of strength endurance, vitality, and energy. Of course, any good cardio program will do that. However, I intend to provide an awesome cardio routine for you to implement that will maximize the most out of your time, keep things interesting and spare your joints.

There's no better way to make a routine low-impact than with the elliptical. If you have not had the luxury of using an elliptical, I highly advise you do so right away. This piece of equipment gets sweat out of you efficiently and trains your heart effectively. All while nurturing your joints from constant banging and rattling that you'd normally have from cardio-based programming.

Whenever I workout on an elliptical, it's my intent to push it to its breaking point. You not only see me working the machine hard, but you can hear me too. I whip the hell out of the elliptical, hence *The Elliptical Whippin' Routine*.

Pictured below is the elliptical that I used for programming. Now, that is not to say that you cannot use this routine with a different elliptical. Just make the necessary modifications in the programming to suit the different brand or type of elliptical.

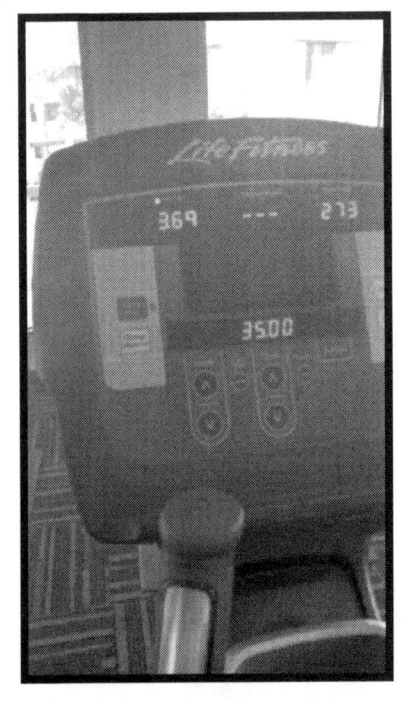

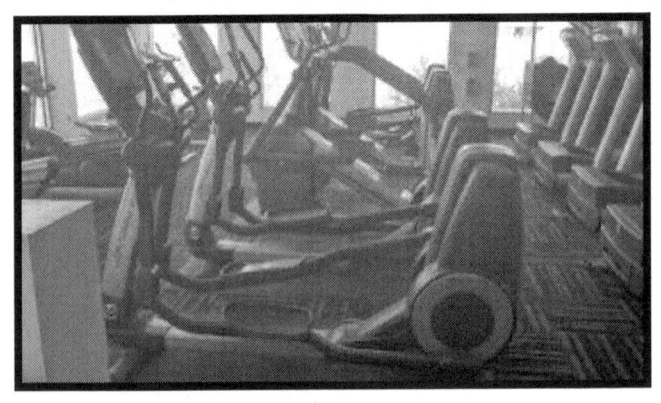

The 11 Best Cardio Workouts

Part 2.1: *Elliptical Whippin'*

MINUTE	LEVEL	PACE
0-5	5	6.0-6.5
5-6	6	10sec. @ 14.0-15.0, 10sec. @ 3.0 (repeat x2)
6-7	4	6.0-6.5
7-8	5	15sec. @ 14.0-15.0, 15sec. @ 3.0 (repeat)
8-9	7	6.0-6.5
9-10	6	20sec. @ 14.0-15.0, 20sec. @ 3.0, 20sec. @ 14.0-15.0
10-15	8	6.0-6.5
15-16	7	30sec. @ 14.0-15.0, 30sec. @ 3.0
16-17	9	6.0-6.5
17-18	8	10sec. @ 14.0-15.0, 10sec. @ 3.0 (repeat x2)
18-19	10	6.0-6.5
19-20	9	15sec. @ 14.0-15.0, 15sec. @ 3.0 (repeat)
20-21	11	6.0-6.5
21-22	10	20sec. @ 14.0-15.0, 20sec. @ 3.0, 20sec. @ 14.0-15.0
22-23	12	6.0-6.5
23-24	11	30sec. @ 14.0-15.0, 30sec. @ 3.0
24-25	13	6.0-6.5
25-26	12	10sec. @ 14.0-15.0, 10sec. @ 3.0 (repeat x2)
26-27	14	6.0-6.5
27-28	13	15sec. @ 14.0-15.0, 15sec. @ 3.0 (repeat)
28-29	15	6.0-6.5
29-30	14	20sec. @ 14.0-15.0, 20sec. @ 3.0, 20sec. @ 14.0-15.0
30-35	-	Pre-programmed cooldown

Part 2.2: Elliptical Whippin'

Continuing on from the first part of *Elliptical Whippin'*, I have an excellent progression that brings your heart rate training to an all new level.

The 11 Best Cardio Workouts

MINUTE	LEVEL	PACE
0-5	5	6.0-6.5
5-6	6	10sec. @ 14.0-15.0, 10sec. @ 3.0 (repeat x2)
6-7	4	6.0-6.5
7-8	5	15sec. @ 14.0-15.0, 15sec. @ 3.0 (repeat)
8-9	7	6.0-6.5
9-10	6	30sec. @ 14.0-15.0, 30sec. @ 3.0
10-15	8	6.0-6.5
15-16	7	14.0-15.0
16-17	9	6.0-6.5
17-18	8	10sec. @ 14.0-15.0, 10sec. @ 3.0 (repeat x2)
18-19	10	6.0-6.5
19-20	9	15sec. @ 14.0-15.0, 15sec. @ 3.0 (repeat)
20-21	11	6.0-6.5
21-22	10	30sec. @ 14.0-15.0, 30sec. @ 3.0
22-23	12	6.0-6.5
23-24	11	14.0-15.0
24-25	13	6.0-6.5
25-26	12	10sec. @ 14.0-15.0, 10sec. @ 3.0 (repeat x2)
26-27	14	6.0-6.5
27-28	13	15sec. @ 14.0-15.0, 15sec. @ 3.0 (repeat)
28-29	15	6.0-6.5
29-30	14	30sec. @ 14.0-15.0, 30sec. @ 3.0
30-35	-	Pre-programmed cooldown

Part 2.3: Elliptical Whippin'

Anyone who says cardio is boring is freaking wrong and this third part in the series is no exception to the rule. The levels continually increase without any recession for the entire workout, so proceed with caution. Do your best and slow your pace should it become too difficult. Remember, do not progress to this routine until you have mastered the first two routines. Enjoy!

The 11 Best Cardio Workouts

MINUTE	LEVEL	PACE
0-5	5	6.0-6.5
5-6	6	10sec. @ 14.0-15.0, 10sec. @ 3.0 (repeat x2)
6-7	6	6.0-6.5
7-8	7	15sec. @ 14.0-15.0, 15sec. @ 3.0 (repeat)
8-9	7	6.0-6.5
9-10	8	20sec. @ 14.0-15.0, 20sec. @ 3.0, 20sec. @ 14.0-15.0
10-15	8	6.0-6.5
15-16	9	30sec. @ 14.0-15.0, 30sec. @ 3.0
16-17	9	6.0-6.5
17-18	10	10sec. @ 14.0-15.0, 10sec. @ 3.0 (repeat x2)
18-19	10	6.0-6.5
19-20	11	15sec. @ 14.0-15.0, 15sec. @ 3.0 (repeat)
20-21	11	6.0-6.5
21-22	12	20sec. @ 14.0-15.0, 20sec. @ 3.0, 20sec. @ 14.0-15.0
22-23	12	6.0-6.5
23-24	13	30sec. @ 14.0-15.0, 30sec. @ 3.0
24-25	13	6.0-6.5
25-26	14	10sec. @ 14.0-15.0, 10sec. @ 3.0 (repeat x2)
26-27	14	6.0-6.5
27-28	15	15sec. @ 14.0-15.0, 15sec. @ 3.0 (repeat)
28-29	15	6.0-6.5
29-30	16	20sec. @ 14.0-15.0, 20sec. @ 3.0, 20sec. @ 14.0-15.0
30-35	-	Pre-programmed cooldown

Part 2.4: Elliptical Whippin'

If this chapter were a house, then part one laid the foundation and part two put up the framework. Part three set up the walls and now we're about to put a roof on this house to make it whole. Proceed with caution.

The 11 Best Cardio Workouts

MINUTES	LEVEL	PACE
0-5	5	6.0-6.5
5-6	6	10sec. @ 14.0-15.0, 10sec. @ 3.0 (repeat x2)
6-7	6	6.0-6.5
7-8	7	15sec. @ 14.0-15.0, 15sec. @ 3.0 (repeat)
8-9	7	6.0-6.5
9-10	8	30sec. @ 14.0-15.0, 30sec. @ 3.0
10-15	8	6.0-6.5
15-16	9	14.0-15.0
16-17	9	6.0-6.5
17-18	10	10sec. @ 14.0-15.0, 10sec. @ 3.0 (repeat x2)
18-19	10	6.0-6.5
19-20	11	15sec. @ 14.0-15.0, 15sec. @ 3.0 (repeat)
20-21	11	6.0-6.5
21-22	12	30sec. @ 14.0-15.0, 30sec. @ 3.0
22-23	12	6.0-6.5
23-24	13	14.0-15.0
24-25	13	6.0-6.5
25-26	14	10sec. @ 14.0-15.0, 10sec. @ 3.0 (repeat x2)
26-27	14	6.0-6.5
27-28	15	15sec. @ 14.0-15.0, 15sec. @ 3.0 (repeat)
28-29	15	6.0-6.5
29-30	16	30sec. @ 14.0-15.0, 30sec. @ 3.0
30-35	-	Pre-programmed cooldown

Dale L. Roberts

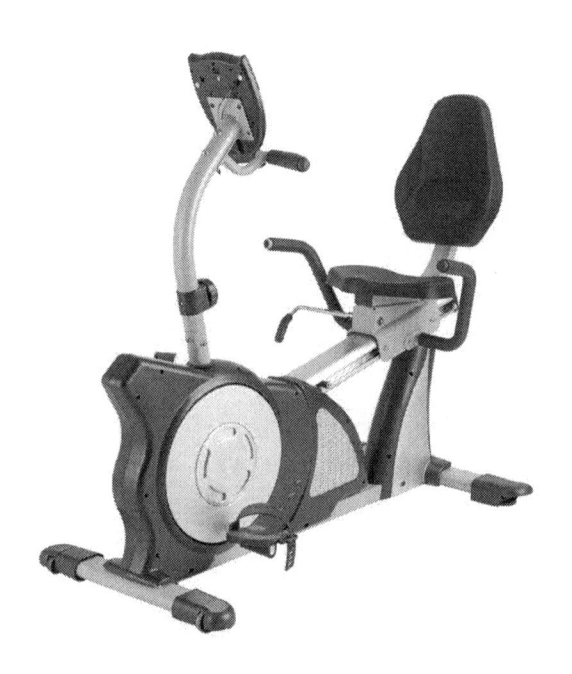

The Four Break-a-bike Routines

You may be missing out on a piece of cardio equipment that could revolutionize your training. A lot of people focus on the treadmill, the elliptical and sometimes the stepmill, but one of the greatest tools in your cardio toolbox lies in the recumbent bike. If you focus on your intensity, you will break a great sweat and get your heart rate up in no time.

An inside joke I have with my wife is that every time we step into the gym, we try to break the cardio equipment. Now, that's not to say we literally destroy it, rather that we push ourselves heavily so that you hear our efforts across the room as the equipment cries from our punishing pace. Hence, the title of the recumbent bike routine—break-a-bike. Please don't try to break cardio equipment, because I cannot be held responsible for broken equipment or paying your hospital bills from hurting yourself in your workout.

With three different recumbent bike routines, you have a variety of choices to fight boredom while training your heart. They are increasingly harder, so master each cardio program in order of first to last. Now, whoop that bike and have some fun!

Part 3.1: Break-a-bike

TIME	LEVEL	RPM
0-5	5	80
5-6	7	>110
6-7	6	80
7-8	8	>110
8-9	7	80
9-10	9	>110
10-11	8	80
11-12	10	>110
12-13	9	80
13-14	11	>110
14-15	10	80
15-16	12	>110
16-17	11	80
17-18	13	>110
18-19	12	80
19-20	14	>110
20-21	13	80
21-22	15	>110
22-23	14	80
23-24	16	>110
24-25	15	80
25-30	5	60

Part 3.2: Break-a-bike

The first bike workout was a primer—something to get you completely ready for the next two weeks. Many cardio routines exist out there, but few focus on the recumbent bike like this program. This cardio program will get you huffing and puffing in the first 10 minutes.

TIME	LEVEL	RPM
0-5	5	80
5-9	5	20 seconds @ 110, 10 seconds @ 80
9-10	5	80
10-14	6	20 seconds @ 110, 10 seconds @ 60, REPEAT
14-15	6	80
15-19	7	20 seconds @ 110, 10 seconds @ 60, REPEAT
19-20	7	80
20-24	8	30 seconds @ 110, 30 seconds @ 80
24-25	8	80
25-30	5	60

Part 3.3: Break-a-bike

As per usual, do not progress to this final routine before you have mastered the first two Break-a-bike routines.

The 11 Best Cardio Workouts

TIME	LEVEL	RPM
0-5	5	80
5-6	10	30 seconds @ 110, 30 seconds @ 80
6-7	9	30 seconds @ 110, 30 seconds @ 80
7-8	8	30 seconds @ 110, 30 seconds @ 80
8-9	7	30 seconds @ 110, 30 seconds @ 80
9-10	6	30 seconds @ 110, 30 seconds @ 80
10-11	5	80
11-12	15	30 seconds @ 110, 30 seconds @ 80
12-13	13	30 seconds @ 110, 30 seconds @ 80
13-14	11	30 seconds @ 110, 30 seconds @ 80
14-15	9	30 seconds @ 110, 30 seconds @ 80
15-16	7	30 seconds @ 110, 30 seconds @ 80
16-17	5	80
17-18	15	30 seconds @ 110, 30 seconds @ 80
18-19	12	30 seconds @ 110, 30 seconds @ 80
19-20	9	30 seconds @ 110, 30 seconds @ 80
20-21	6	30 seconds @ 110, 30 seconds @ 80
21-22	5	80
22-23	15	30 seconds @ 110, 30 seconds @ 80
23-24	11	30 seconds @ 110, 30 seconds @ 80
24-25	7	30 seconds @ 110, 30 seconds @ 80
25-30	5	60

Conclusion

Working out and getting in shape should not be a drag. Exercising needs to be fun, engaging and something you look forward to every day. This book is merely a snapshot and only eleven options in an ocean of choices to better your health. If you choose to use these routines, do it to the best of your abilities. However, in the event you didn't find value in it, don't stop looking for options that work for you. Many excellent options for cardio training include:

1. -Running
2. -Hiking
3. -Biking
4. -Dancing
5. -Group fitness classes
6. -Weight training
7. -And, so much more!

Remember to always have 16-32 ounce of water for during your cardio workout. And, drink an additional 16-32 ounces of water after your workout. Hydration is crucial to getting the most out of your workout. You will sweat a lot throughout your workout, so replenish all of your bodily fluids with plenty of water. Dehydration is a setback you do not want to experience, so do your best to drink water frequently and abundantly.

A small yet worth investment is a heart rate monitor. Some cardio equipment comes with heart rate monitors, but sometimes they do not

The 11 Best Cardio Workouts

function properly. Owning a heart rate monitor will have you covered for all your workouts, regardless of the equipment have a working monitor or not. A good heart rate monitor helps you focus your efforts specific to your fitness levels and goals. This fitness tool tells you when you are working too hard or not hard enough.

Depending on your health and fitness goals, you may want to do a minimum of one cardio session per week. If you are new to cardio training, ease your way into doing three sessions per week and do not exceed more than five of these cardio sessions in one week. If you are more experienced, then you should have the capacity to gauge the number of cardio workouts you can handle per week.

In closing, for those of you struggling with your weight or having issues with finding the right fitness routine for you—don't give up. Whatever you do, remember that the reward of greater health and wellness is far better than the risks that being overweight or obesity brings. Cardio should be fun and it's my hope that I provided you the right solution. In the event, I didn't, keep searching and trying until you get it right. When you find discouragement, remember that other people walked your path before and can help you get through tough times. Don't be afraid to bring a friend along to make workouts more engaging. Hire a personal trainer or find a mentor who can show you the way. And, always lead by great example for the other people just like you, because you never know who is watching. You may not only change your life, but you may positively affect the world around you. Now get out there and get your heart in shape!

Thank You

Thank you for taking the time to read my book. I hope that you enjoyed reading it as much as I enjoyed writing it. I have only one request; if you did like it, please leave a review. Reviews are the lifeblood of indie and small press authors and greatly help us get more books in front of more readers. If you didn't like it, that's fine too. Just leave an honest review, that's all I ask. Drop me a review on Amazon.com.

As you work toward your goals, you may have questions or run into some issues. I'd like to be able to help you, so let's connect. I don't charge for the assistance, so feel free to connect with me on the internet at:

DaleLRoberts.com
Like me on Facebook:
http://www.facebook.com/authordaleroberts
Follow me on Twitter:
@ptdaleroberts
Subscribe to my YouTube channel:
http://www.youtube.com/ptdalelroberts

Thank you, again! I hope to hear from you and wish you the best.
-Dale

P.S. You will find my entire catalog of books on Amazon Author Central at amazon.com/author/daleroberts. Click the "Follow" button to get updates any time I publish a new book.

About The Author

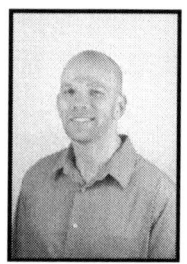

My name is Dale Lewis Roberts and I'm an American Council on Exercise Personal Trainer, Certified, with an ACE Specialty Certification in Senior Fitness. Since beginning my personal training career in 2006, I have earned numerous certifications in personal training, yoga, nutritional coaching, among others. I have worked with hundreds of clients with a variety of health & fitness goals.

While my greatest passions are health & fitness, writing and reading, I also love to spend time traveling with my wife, watching pro wrestling and playing guitar. I currently reside in Phoenix, Arizona, with my wife, Kelli, and our rescue cat, Izzie.

Subscribe to my blog at <u>DaleLRoberts.com</u> for all the latest posts on health and fitness tips. This is also one of the best ways to connect with me directly. Please, remember that whatever you do in life, make sure that you do what you love. Stay happy, healthy and strong!

Special Thanks

As always, I have my deepest gratitude for the love of my life, Kelli. You are the reason I stay up extra late and wake up extra early just so I have the chance to make you proud. And, I owe a debt of gratitude to my mentor and friend, Jason Bracht. You bring out the best in me and challenge me to provide my reading audience nothing but the best. Lastly, Sami Johnston, I appreciate your selfless efforts and time into developing my branding. You are the man!

__ATTENTION: Get Your Free Gift__

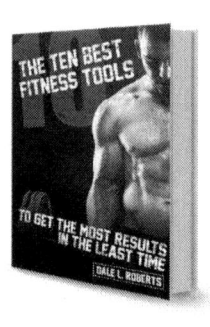

Are you interested in learning about the ten best fitness tools in fat loss? You are not alone! Millions of people all over the world are trying to lose weight and do so in a safe and effective manner.

What I have done is put together a FREE report to get you started on the road to success. This report won't be up forever, so get them before they are taken down. It's my simple way of saying thank you for buying this book.

http://DaleLRoberts.com/tenbest

Download the report on "The Ten Best Fitness Tools (To Get You More Results in the Least Time)" ABSOLUTELY FREE. The tips in this report will help you lose weight, melt off fat, and get in great shape!

References

[i] Brainy Quote. (n.d.). Benjamin Franklin Quotes. Retrieved on 2015, October 14 from http://www.brainyquote.com/quotes/quotes/b/benjaminfr129817.html

[ii] World Health Organization. (2015, January). Obesity and overweight – Fact Sheet N° 311. Retrieved from http://www.who.int/mediacentre/factsheets/fs311/en/

[iii] Kravitz, Len. (2014). High-Intensity Interval Training. Retrieved on 2105, October 15 from https://www.acsm.org/docs/brochures/high-intensity-interval-training.pdf

[iv] Harvard Men's Health Watch. (2002, January 11). Maximum heart rate: A new formula for fitness. Retrieved from https://portal.yafferuden.com/html/maximum_heartrate.html

Made in the USA
Lexington, KY
20 April 2016